A Grief-stricken Mind

A Shocking Reality of How Humans Learn from Love and Death

Jackie L. Schatz

All rights reserved. No part of this publication may be reproduced, distributed, or transmitted in any form or by any means, including photocopying, recording, or other electronic or mechanical methods, without the prior written permission of the publisher, except in the case of brief quotations embodied in critical reviews and certain other noncommercial uses permitted by copyright law.

Copyright © by **Jackie L. Schatz 2022**

Table of content

After someone we love passes away, holidays are never the same.

Even the smallest details of a birthday or Christmas celebration — an empty place at the dinner table, one less gift to buy or manufacture — can serve as stark reminders of how drastically our lives have changed.

It's difficult to adjust to the realization that we'll never see our loved ones again.

It takes time, and it requires brain changes.

"What we observe in science is that if you have a mourning experience and have support so that you have some time to learn and confidence from others around you, you can recover."

When we have the experience of being in a relationship, we associate our sense of ourselves with the other person. The words brother and spouse both imply two persons. As a result, when the other person leaves, we are forced to learn a completely new set of norms in order to function in the world. The "we" is just as crucial as the "you" and "me," and the brain actually encodes it that way. It's for this reason that many say "I feel like I've lost a piece of myself."

On the distinction between grief and mourning

Grief is an emotional state that sweeps you off your feet and sweeps you off your feet. Grieving is inextricably linked to the passage of time. Grieving is the process of adjusting to the fact that our loved one is no longer with us, that we are carrying their absence with us. And the reason for this distinction is that grieving is a natural reaction to loss, thus we'll always be sad. Because it's a new moment where she's having a response to loss, a lady who lost her mother as a child will experience that sadness on her wedding day.
However, "grieving" implies that our reaction to loss evolves through time. So the first time, possibly the first time,

On long-term grief

"When will this end?" you wonder as you're knocked over by the flood of grief. According to research, a very small percentage of people may develop what is now known as extended mourning disorder, which we check for after six months or a year [after a death or loss]. And what we're seeing here is that this person hasn't been able to perform as well as they would like daily. They can't get out the door to work or put dinner on the table for their children, or they can't listen to music because it's too upsetting. As a result, these kinds of worries indicate it.

"Complicated grief" was an older word that we used for a long time. Although we've landed on the phrase "prolonged grief disorder," I like the term "complex" because it conjures up images of problems.

One of the most difficult tasks that many of us encounter are dealing with the loss of a close friend or family member. Although loss is accepted as a normal part of life, we can nevertheless be struck with shock and bewilderment, leading to persistent melancholy or depression. Although the sadness usually fades with time, grieving is a vital step in overcoming these emotions and continuing to cherish the time you had with your loved one.

Everyone handles death differently and has their own grief coping techniques. Most people may recover from loss on their own over time if they have social support and good behaviours, according to research. Expect to go through phases of mourning as well, as research shows that most people do not go through them in sequential order.

If your relationship with the deceased was strained, the grieving process will be complicated further. It may take some time and consideration before you can reflect on the connection and adjust to the loss.

Humans are innately resilient, as evidenced by the fact that most of us can survive loss and go on with our lives. However, other people may experience grief for extended periods and find themselves unable to carry out regular tasks. Individuals experiencing severe or complex sorrow may benefit from the assistance of a psychologist or another certified mental health practitioner who specializes in grief.

Accept your emotions.

All of these emotions are normal, and it's critical to recognize them as they arise. If you're feeling stuck or overwhelmed by these sentiments, speaking with a certified psychologist or another mental health expert can help you cope with your emotions and find solutions to get back on track.

Allow yourself to heal.

Moving on from a painful or difficult event, such as a breakup or the death of a loved one, takes time. Don't put too much pressure on yourself to let go or move on before you're ready. Allow yourself to experience your sadness, anger, or anxiety as it arises, and remember that you will not always feel the same way.

You'll undoubtedly have ups and downs after a defeat or any other tough experience. Don't be disheartened if you start to feel better one day and then start suffering the next.

Part 2

The majority of us have a proclivity to dwell in the past or the future. How often do you find yourself reflecting on what occurred yesterday or what might occur tomorrow? What impact does this have on your life and health?

In this post, we'll talk about how to live in the present moment more often and some strategies for resuming mindful living.

Take in Your Environment...

Observing your environment is one approach to being in the present moment. When was the last time you sat down, closed your eyes, took a deep breath, and simply observe your surroundings?

What are your thoughts on the walls?
What about designs on the

floor or ceiling?
To your left and right, how
many windows do you have?

How many lights can you
count from this vantage point?

It's simpler to live in the
present moment when you take
a moment to glance around
and take in everything around
you.

Be Thankful For What You
Already Have...

Taking the time to be grateful for what you have today is an important part of living in the present moment (not in the past or the future).

Writing a list of things, you are grateful for and reviewing it on a daily basis is one approach to practicing gratitude. Write down at least three things you are grateful for right now in your life.

Meditation for Mindfulness

Please take a seat. Find a seat that gives you a sturdy, solid seat, not perching or hanging back, whether it's a chair, a meditation cushion, or a park bench.
Take note of how your legs are moving. (If you're already in a seated yoga position, go ahead.) If you're sitting on a chair, the bottoms of your feet

should be touching the floor.

Straighten your upper body without stiffening it. Natural curvature exists in the spine. Allow it to exist.

Feel (or "follow") your breath as it leaves and enters your body. (Some variations of this technique emphasize the out-breath while leaving a spacious interval for the in-breath.) In any case, focus on the physical feeling of breathing: air going through your nose or mouth, your abdomen rising and falling, or your chest rising and falling. Choose a focal point and mentally note "breathing in" and "breathing

out" with each breath. Your attention will inevitably leave the breath and stray to other things. Don't be concerned. There is no need to stop or stop thinking. When

you see your mind
wandering—in a few seconds,
a minute, five minutes—return
your focus to it gently.

If you believe in empowerment, ownership, authenticity, and transparency, it's time to quit believing that our sentiments are caused by other people or things.
1) the distinction between affect and emotion

2) Recognizing how we place blame on others for our emotions

3) avoiding emotional classifications based on myths

4) Putting the five steps for emotional accountability into action.

Assume you're driving to work and passing through your neighbourhood coffee shop's drive-through. The queue is quite long, and it is moving quite slowly today. You have a crucial presentation to make to your team today, and you have a meeting in a few minutes. You overhear an older woman in front of you asking a lot of questions about the menu, attempting to understand the difference between an iced coffee and a cold brew. They take a long time to make up their minds. What are your thoughts?

Assume you're in the same drive-through, but you're driving on a camping trip with your daughter. You're with her, and you're talking about how much fun you're going to have at the lake. You don't have a set schedule, you have the entire weekend ahead of you, and you're with one of your favourite people. You overhear an older person in front of you asking a lot of questions about the menu, attempting to figure out what the difference is between an iced coffee and a cold brew.

What are your thoughts on the situation?

Consider your emotions in both circumstances and respond to the following question: "Where did your emotions come from?" What made you feel that way? Who is to blame for how you are feeling right now?

Emotion vs. Affect

The forces that precede, produce, and inform our experiences are known as effects. The effect is not personal or subjective; it is the product of external forces acting on us. Affect is the pre-subjective experience we get as a result of the situational elements in the scenarios above; for example, a lengthy line, a sluggish order ahead of you, the clock ticking, and your daughter sitting next to you. The effect isn't so much what you feel as it is what makes you feel. Affect frequently entails an unconscious physiological response, such as a faster heart rate or stomach butterflies.

Your emotions are the product of how you interact with the world around you and within yourself. They're the product of your one-of-a-kind encounter. As seen by the instances above, two people witnessing the same external situation can have the same influence but exhibit distinct feelings. Nobody or nothing has the power to make you feel a specific way.

Emotional Responsibility in Three Steps

It's fine to name your feelings,

give them a name, and express them honestly.

Rather than looking for someone or something to blame, go yourself and accept responsibility for how you came to your emotion.

It's fine to challenge inappropriate behaviour, but don't blame people for your emotions.

Keep an eye on everything you do.

You should be aware of everything you do, from eating to looking through your phone. How often do you eat your lunch while also watching TV? This is one way to detach yourself from what you're doing and avoid living in the present moment because your full concentration isn't focused on it.

Instead, try to concentrate on each meal while you eat it. What is the aroma of the food? What does it taste like? How is your body responding to the food you've consumed so far? What sounds are there while you are eating - phone calls, outside road noises, background music? By concentrating on these things and becoming aware of them,

Taking a break from social media and other forms of technology might also help you focus on the present. While you may believe that checking your social media accounts regularly keeps you connected to the world, it hinders your capacity to be present.

How many times have you found yourself checking social media while doing anything else? You must understand how to avoid allowing technology to take over your life because this can cause you to lose track of what's going on around you.

It's critical to be aware of how you use social media to guarantee that it has a beneficial impact on your health. That involves understanding when to go away and focus on something else.

Keep in mind that using social media is a sedentary activity. Even if you're talking to friends, social media reduces your ability for face-to-face contacts, causing you to spend less time outside and more time on your phone or computer. Furthermore, if you find yourself comparing other people's lives to your own, social media may induce tension, worry, or despair.

"In terms of mental health," Katara McCarty, founder of EXHALE, a well-being app for Black and Indigenous Women of Color, explains, "social media can influence our self-esteem and lead to us comparing ourselves to altered photographs and lives that appear flawless." "We aren't taking the time to take care of our bodies and enjoy life outside of social media if we spend long periods on social media."

You might want to be somewhere else while you're experiencing the burn.

Apart from the gym, everywhere. Your body, on the other hand, is thanking you for the entire time; exercise has profound impacts on both the body and the mind.

www.ingramcontent.com/pod-product-compliance
Lightning Source LLC
Chambersburg PA
CBHW052136150726
48002CB00006B/2636